Vegan Diet

14 Days Meal Plans and Everyday Recipes with Calories and Macronutrients for Each Meal for Beginners

(A Simple and Fast Vegan Cookbook)

Rusty Bond

Published by Robert Satterfield
Publishing House

© **Rusty Bond**

All Rights Reserved

Vegan Diet: 14 Days Meal Plans and Everyday Recipes with Calories and Macronutrients for Each Meal for Beginners (A Simple and Fast Vegan Cookbook)

ISBN 978-1-989682-87-6

Legal & Disclaimer

The information contained in this book is not designed to replace or take the place of any form of medicine or professional medical advice. The information in this book has been provided for educational and entertainment purposes only.

TABLE OF CONTENT

Part 1

33 Simple Vegan Recipes for Beginners

Disclaimer

NO ANIMALS WERE HARMED IN THE MAKING OF THIS BOOK.

Not sure what vegan food can do for you?

Look, I get it. You're a little V-curious like me. Maybe you just watched one of those shocking yet eye-opening documentaries like Earthlings or Cowspiracy. Maybe your friend from your

yoga class has told you she's eating a plant-based diet from now on and you want to know

what the heck it's all about. Countless times I've heard people bash vegan food for being unhealthy, lacking in nutrients and being downright disgusting. Don't worry. They are wrong.

Vegan food can be incredibly delicious and rich in everything your body needs.

If you're just starting out with veganism, you don't have to go cold-turkey from day one (if you have turkey left in your fridge, don't throw it out, okay?). Finish your non-vegan stuff you have at home, or give it to your friends or neighbors if you real y can't stand it anymore.

Don't throw food in the bin, though. That's just unnecessary and bad for the planet. It's fine to just take it slow and ditch your bacon and cheese only every other day. Do things in your own pace. Maybe keep one meal per day completely free of animal products and go on from

there. Why not start with the most important meal of the day, breakfast, and fil it with plant-based goodness?

Got no idea how to get started? This book will sort you out! But first, let's recap the reasons why people choose to give animal products the boot (leather-free)

Vegan for the Animals

How often do you think about where your food comes from? Before every meal my parents

say grace and praise the Lord for the food he's put on their table. But that's not where their Bratwurst has come from. It's not the Almighty who's handing them their slab of beef, it's the friendly neighborhood butcher. And before that the meat was an actual live animal, who

didn't live happily ever after. It was kil ed, and if it's not from some magical place in the far away Mongolian grasslands, it was probably raised in a factory farm and slaughtered by

slitting its throat. If you've seen one of those gruesome undercover videos taken in factory farms and slaughterhouses, you know what I'm talking about. It's not nice. Not at all. So why support that?

But what about milk and cheese? That's cool, ain't it? Wel , have you ever seen those breast pumps for mothers that can't breastfeed their babies? Imagine strapping those onto the next woman you see and locking her into a cage. Then you force her to … okay, I'm gonna stop

here. Please don't do that. But you get the picture, right? Dairy production is cruel as sh*t.

And given that the cows are being kept pregnant almost all the time, then have their calves taken from their care way too early, and are constantly being forced to produce milk until they're too old and weak, one could argue that dairy production is actual y worse from an ethical point of view than meat production. Jesus, I real y want to jump to those awesome vegan banana pancakes now, but bear with me, if you like.

Vegan for the Planet

Are you ready for some numbers? Alrighty, let's go! In 2017, animal agriculture for food production - also called livestock - caused about 14.5% of global emissions of greenhouse

gases, which is more than the whole transportation sector [1]. Greenhouse gases, by the way, are the driving force behind human-induced climate change and global warming. Now,

unless you're thinking "Oh, I like it nice and warm and hurricany", this should concern you a wee bit. But even if it doesn't, animal agriculture has more adverse effects on the

environment. Raising livestock uses about 70% of agricultural land and causes loss of

biodiversity, deforestation and pollution of water [1].

As you can see, raising animals for our consumption uses large amounts of land and

resources and has dire impacts on the environment (think about those cow farts!). You don't have to be a genius to see the only possible solution. Cutting down on animal products in our diet can help combating climate change and making a positive shift towards a

sustainable future.

Vegan for your Body

Okay, if the stuff about the animals and the environment hasn't sold you yet, maybe this one wil do the trick. Despite what many people believe, a vegan diet can have positive effects on your health. A vegan is sometimes depicted as a scrawny and sickly looking dude with

dreadlocks and a tie-dye shirt. But that cliché is a thing from the past. Just check out the bodybuilder and calisthenics expert Frank Medrano. That guy is shredded as hell and strong like a T-1000 Terminator. Do you think this is only possible with a diet fil ed with chicken, fish oil and loads of whey protein shakes? Wrong. Frank is 100% plant powered and living proof that you can kil it in the gym on a vegan diet.

In fact, vegans tend to be thinner than their meat eating counterpart, have lower serum

cholesterol and blood pressure, which in return reduces their risk of heart disease [2]. While a well-balanced diet containing all the required nutrients is always important, going vegan can give your body the extra health-boost it needs.

A little disclaimer at the end: If you're unsure that your body can thrive on a vegan diet, please contact your doctor and ask for actual medical advice. Alternatively you could reduce your intake of animal products to a minimum but stil eat meat or something else from time to time to be on the safe side. But yeah, if you're going the full V, please consult a doctor first.

I'm not a professional and everything presented in this book is for informational purposes only. There, now that we have that out of the way, let's move on to the meat of this book (pun intended). Ladies and gentlemen, may I present to you...

The Recipes

Part I: Breakfast

Recipe 1 - OMFG Oatmeal

Let's start our journey with a real classic. This oatmeal is easy absolutely yummy!

The Ingredients (1 Serving)

- ½ cup rolled oats

- 1 cup of water

- 1 pinch of salt

- 1 pinch of cinnamon

- 3.5 oz blueberries

- ½ fresh apple, diced (Granny Smith or any other "green" apple)

- 3 TSP crushed almonds or hazelnuts

The Instructions

1. Mix the water with the oats in a saucepan and add the salt and cinnamon. Boil that

stuff then bring the heat down again. Watch out that you don't burn it.

2. Let the mix simmer without a lid for about 3-4 minutes. Stir gently from time to time and watch as the plot... err... the oatmeal thickens. Remove the pan from the heat

and let it all cool down a bit.

3. Fil the yummy goodness into a bowl and top it off with the blueberries, the apple

dices and the crushed almond or nuts (and whatever floats your boat, real y)

4. ENJOY

Recipe 2 - You Pancake, I Banana

Final y! It's time for pancakes. No, you don't need eggs for them. Ripe bananas work just fine and give the pancakes a yummy taste on top!

The Ingredients (1 Serving)

● ½ cup of blanched almond flour

● 1 small but very ripe banana

● ¼ cup of almond or soy milk

● 2 tablespoons baking powder

● 2 tablespoons vegetable oil

● 1 tablespoon brown sugar (white sugar is also okay)

● 1 pinch of salt

● 1 tablespoon puffed amaranth (optional for more fluffiness)

● 1 pinch of cinnamon (optional but yummy)

- Optional toppings: maple sirup; cinnamon & sugar; soy yogurt

The Instructions

1. Mix the flour, sugar, salt and baking powder in a bowl. Mash the banana and stir it in together with the almond milk and vegetable oil until the mixture is thoroughly

combined. Optional: If you like the pancakes extra fluffy, you can try to find some

puffed amaranth and add 1 tablespoon to the mix.

2. Heat a small to medium-sized frying pan over medium heat. You could even get

some of those awesome cast iron pancake pans. Finding the right heat can be a pain

as it depends totally on your stove and pans. But with a little practice you'l find your sweet spot quickly.

3. Drop a large spoonful of pancake batter onto the pan and make sure the batter is

wel distributed. Within 2 to 3 minutes bubbles should pop and the surface of the

pancake becomes matte. Then you know it's time to flip over. Cook the other side for

another 2 minutes.

4. Place the finished pancake on a plate and repeat the previous steps with the

remaining batter. Once al pancakes are ready, add the topping of your preference. I

love pancake with plain old cinnamon and sugar, but you might be a sucker for maple

sirup. Or just have it all!

5. Enjoy!

Recipe 3 - The Power Sandwich RAWWRR

It doesn't get simpler that this. But the sandwich is stil mega tasty and super nutricious!

The Ingredients (1 Serving)

• 2 slices of toast (preferably sourdough or levain toast)

• ½ avocado

• 1 sweet potato

• 1 red paprika

• 1 tomato

• 2 leaves of lettuce

• a few leaves of parsley

• salt & pepper

• some vegetable oil

The Instructions

1. Before you roast the bread, you need to fry the sweet potato in thin slices. Cut

about four to six slices from the middle of the sweet potato and place the remaining piece

back in your fridge. The slices wil be the meat of your sandwich. Fry them in a pan

with the vegetable oil until they are soft and golden brown on both sides. Flip the

slices in the pan regularly.

2. While the sweet potato slices are gently frying, cut open the avocado and scoop out

one half into a small bowl. Mash the avocado with a fork and add some salt and

pepper. If you're feeling adventurous you can add some chili flakes too.

3. Roast the bread and cut one or two slices of tomato, and a couple of thin rings from

the paprika. Take out the sweet potato from the frying pan and let the slices cool for a

minute.

4. Spread about half of the avocado paste on one slice of roasted bread. Add the

lettuce on top of the avocado paste. Put the sweet potato slices on the lettuce,

followed by the tomato and paprika. Top it off with some salt and pepper, and add the

parsley. This wil give the sandwich an even fresher taste. Spread the remaining

avocado paste on the second slice of bread and complete your sandwich.

5. Enjoy!

Recipe 4 - Better Be Banana Bread

More banana stuff, yay! This bread is soft and goes well with jam or fresh fruit.

The Ingredients (1 Loaf)

- 1 cup oat flour

- ½ cup coconut flour

- 1 tablespoon raw cacao

- 1 teaspoon kanel

- 1 teaspoon bakpulver

- 1/2 teaspoon salt

- 2,5 ripe bananas

- 1 tablespoon coconut oil

- 1 teaspoon vanil a powder

- ⅓ cup almond milk or soy milk

- crushed almonds or hazelnuts as topping

The Instructions

1. Preheat the oven to 400°F (or 200°C).

2. Mash the bananas.

3. Mix all the dry ingredients in a bowl.

4. Add all other ingredients to the mix.

5. If the mix is too runny, add some additional oat flour.

6. Grease the bread pan with some vegan margarine or spread and fil in the dough.

Make sure it's evenly distributed. Add the crushed almonds or hazelnuts on top

7. Place the bread pan on the lowest grill in the oven and bake for about 20 to 30

minutes, depending on your pan and oven. I recommend checking the crust and

consistency inside after 20 minutes.

8. Take out the bread and let it cool down before slicing it.

9. Enjoy with some jam or peanut butter, or both!

Recipe 5 - Get a loaf of this one!

And another bread! This one is also the soft type and can even be enjoyed without a spread thanks to the various nuts and fruits inside.

The Ingredients (1 loaf)

- ¾ cups coconut flour

- 1 cup oat flour

- 1 ½ cups of lukewarm water

- 1 medium sized red apple, grated

- 2 small carrots, grated

- ½ cup raisins

- 2 tablespoons olive oil

- ½ cup crushed hazelnuts

- ½ cup sunflower seeds

- ½ cup linseeds

- 1 ½ tablespoons psyl ium husk powder

- 1 ½ tablespoons psyl ium husk seeds

• 2 teaspoons salt

• 2 ½ teaspoons bicarbonate or baking soda

• 1 tablespoon of apple cider vinegar

The Instructions

1. Preheat oven to 425°F (or 220°C).

2. Mix the dry ingredients in a bowl.

3. Mix the water, the oil and vinegar, the raisins, the grated apple and carrots in another bowl.

4. Pour the dry mix into the bowl of liquids and stir quickly until you have an even but sticky batter. Let it stand for about 10 minutes. The batter will rise during that time.

5. Fil the batter into a bread pan or baking form and cover the surface with some

additional oat flour. Now it's time for the oven. Bake for about 80 minutes.

6. Take out the bread from the form and let it cool down under a kitchen towel before

slicing it.

7. Enjoy your slice of heaven. This should last you a couple of breakfasts!

Recipe 6 - Scramble my Feggs

Alright, I know, I know. Enough of that sweet stuff. I'm also more of a savory breakfast kind of person. And who knew that tofu can be transformed into fake scrambled eggs that not

only look the same as the original, but are just as tasty!

The Ingredients (1 Serving)

• 70 g medium hard tofu

• 50 g silken tofu

• 1 tablespoon vegetable oil

- ½ teaspoon turmeric

- salt & pepper

The Instructions

1. Oil the pan and heat it up slowly to medium heat.

2. Crush the tofu in the pan with a fork until it has the desired size for your fake

scrambled eggs.

3. Season the tofu bits with the turmeric until everything is nice a yellow like real

scrambled eggs. Add some salt and pepper and fry the tofu for about 5 minutes.

4. Enjoy with some avocado on toast, and some fresh parsley on top.

Recipe 7 - I'd like ze Müsli bitte

I've got a German in me, so I have to mention Müsli. Healthy cereals for the win. Forget cornflakes and chocolate puffs and all that sugary crap. Real Müsli is much better for you!

The Ingredients (1 Serving)

● ⅓ cup rolled oats

● 2 tablespoons puffed amaranth

● 2 teaspoons chia seeds

● 3 tablespoons crushed walnuts

● ½ cup soy, almond or oat milk

● 1 kiwi

● ½ apple

● 2 oz raspberries

● 1 pinch of cinnamon

The Instructions

1. Mix the oats, amaranth, chia seeds and crushed walnuts in a bowl.

2. Dice the kiwi and apple half.

3. Add the vegan milk drink of your choice to the dry mix.

4. Add in the fruit and berries and top it all off with a pinch of cinnamon for extra taste.

5. Enjoy ze Müsli like a true German!

Recipe 8 - Smoooothie

Sometimes it's got to go quickly. This smoothie can even be prepared the night before and stored in the fridge over night.

The Ingredients (1 Serving)

- ¾ cups almond/soy/oat milk

- 1 avocado

- 1.5 oz baby spinach

- ½ lemon

- 3.5 oz mango

- 2 teaspoons freshly grated ginger

- 1 teaspoon agave syrup

- 1 tablespoon coconut oil

The Instructions

1. Cut open and carve out the avocado (you can even use the seed to grow your own

avocado tree!).

2. Put all ingredients into a blender. Squeeze in the lemon juice. Blend everything.

3. Pour your smoothie into a glass and top off with some coconut flakes before serving.

4. Enjoy your green goodness!

Recipe 9 - Milk dat rice!

I love milk rice pudding. It's so good with sugar and cinnamon. Here's the vegan variant: The Ingredients (1 Serving)

- 1 cup sticky rice (also goes by the name of glutinous rice)

- 2 cups water

- 1 whole cinnamon stick

- ½ teaspoon salt

- 3 cups almond milk

- 1 teaspoon brown sugar

- 1 pinch cinnamon

The Instructions

1. Fil the water into a pot and add the rice, the cinnamon stick and the salt. Crank up the heat until the water boils. Turn the heat back to medium and cook with the lid

almost covering the whole pot (leave a slight gap on one side). Cook for 10 minutes

without stirring at all.

2. Check if the rice has absorbed all the water. If it has not, continue to cook for a

couple of minutes until all liquid has been absorbed by the rice.

3. Stir in the almond milk thoroughly. Place the lid back on and let the milk rice cook

over low heat for about 40 minutes.

4. Fil the milk rice pudding into a bowl and sprinkle some brown sugar and cinnamon

on top for extra yumminess. Optionally you can add some diced apple.

5. Enjoy!

Recipe 10 - Fruit Woop Salad

Another easy one for lazy people like me. Vitamins, baby!

The Ingredients (1 Serving)

- ½ apple

- 1 oz blackberries

- 1 oz strawberries

- 1 kiwi fruits

- ½ orange

- 1 peach

- 1 oz red grapes, seedless

- 1 oz green grapes, seedless

- ½ lemons

The Instructions

1. Cut the apple, the kiwi and peach into small dice. Peel the fruits before if you like.

2. Wash the grapes and berries, and cut them in halves, or smaller if you want.

3. Put the fruits in a bowl. Squeeze out the orange and lemon halves before adding

their juice to the fruits.

4. Enjoy!

Recipe 11 - Spread This!

If you love bread, you love spread! This yummy spread tastes amazing on fresh sourdough

bread.

The Ingredients (1 Serving)

- 2 tablespoons of sunflower oil

- 1 ¾ oz sunflower seeds

- 1 oz eggplant

- ½ oz lemon juice

- 0.2 oz onions, chopped

- 0.2 oz red bel pepper, chopped

- ⅛ of an apple

- 2 tablespoons of apple juice

- 1 teaspoon of tomato paste

- 1 teaspoon of sugar

- Salt & pepper

- Some basil, oregano and rosemary spices

The Instructions

1. Boil the sunflower seeds in a large pot of water for about 15 minutes. This wil cause the seeds to swell.

2. While the seeds boil, cut the eggplant, apple and bel pepper into thin slices. Gently roast each ingredient in a frying pan.

3. After the seeds have boiled for 15 minutes, pour out the water and mash the seeds

with a hand mixer. Carefully add the juices and the sunflower oil and continue to

blend the mixture until it's nice and creamy.

4. Add the eggplant, apple and bell pepper slices, as well as the tomato paste. Mash and mix some more until you have a creamy spread.

5. Season the spread with salt, pepper, sugar and the other spices.

6. Enjoy the spread on some fresh sourdough bread or baguette. Nom!

The Recipes

Part II: Lunch

Recipe 12 - Lentils, Lime & Curry

Time for lunch! Let's begin with a yummy curry.

The Ingredients (2 Servings)

- 2 portions rice

- ½ cup red lentils, dry

- ½ onion

- 1 garlic clove

- ½ tablespoon fresh ginger, grated

- ½ tablespoon vegetable oil

- ½ teaspoon sambal oelek

- 1 teaspoon tomato paste

- ¼ tablespoon curry

- 1 cup of vegetable broth

- 7 oz coconut milk

- ¼ cauliflower head

- 4 ½ oz cherry tomatoes

- ½ lime

- 1 oz baby spinach

- ⅓ cup cashews, unsalted

- Salt and pepper

The Instructions

1. Boil the rice according to the instructions on the package. I can recommend getting a rice cooker, they rule!

2. Wash the lentils.

3. Peel and dice the onion. Peel and grate the ginger.

4. Gently fry the onion and the sambal oelek in some oil in a big pot. Press the garlic

and stir it in together with the ginger, curry and tomato paste. Add the lentils, the

coconut milk and the vegetable broth. Bring to a boil while stirring continuously, then

let it simmer under a lid for 10 minutes.

5. Cut the cauliflower in smaller bits. Add them in the pot and cook for another 10

minutes.

6. Cut the tomatoes in halves and the lime into wedges.

7. Season the curry with salt and pepper, and stir in the spinach and tomatoes.

8. Serve the lentil curry with rice and top off with lime and cashews.

9. Enjoy!

Recipe 13 - Rice Sweet Chili

Enough of curry? Try some stir fry with sweet chili sauce!

The Ingredients (2 Servings)

- ⅔ cups basmati rice

- ½ carrot

- ½ red bel pepper

- 4 oz sweet peas

- 1 spring onion

- 1 tablespoon vegetable oil

- ¾ tablespoons soy sauce

- 2 tablespoons sweet chili sauce

- Salt and pepper

The Instructions

1. Boil the rice according to the instructions on the package.

2. Peel the carrot. Cut the bell pepper, carrot, sweet peas and spring onion into small

strips.

3. Fry the vegetables with the oil in a wok or big frying pan for about 3 minutes. Season wel with salt and pepper. Add the soy sauce.

4. Add the cooked rice and the sweet chili sauce. Stir thoroughly until everything is well mixed.

5. Serve and enjoy!

Recipe 14 - Rock my Moroccan Carrots

This super easy salad is made quickly and tastes amazing.

The Ingredients (2 Servings)

- 2 lbs baby carrots

- 2 tablespoons olive oil

- 3 garlic cloves

- ¾ cups chopped coriander

- 1 tablespoon freshly pressed lemon juice

- 1 tablespoon harissa spice powder

- 1 teaspoon salt

- 2 teaspoons ground cumin

The Instructions

1. Preheat the oven to 425° F (220° C).

2. Wash the carrots and cut them in long halves. Mix the carrots with the olive oil in a bowl so they're evenly oiled up.

3. Place the carrots on a baking tray and bake them in the middle of the oven for about

15 minutes. The carrots should get a little crispy and brown on the outside and soft in

the middle. Let them cool down afterwards.

4. Dice the garlic cloves. Mix the garlic, the coriander, and the spices with the lemon

juice.

5. Once the carrots have cooled down, mix them with the coriander dressing.

6. Serve and enjoy your healthy and low calorie carrot salad!

Recipe 15 - Chili Sin Carne

A classic made vegan! Good as sin!

The Ingredients (2 Servings)

For the main dish:

- ½ onion

- ½ garlic clove

- ½ red bel pepper

- ½ can of crushed tomatoes

- 1 ½ fresh tomatoes

- 4.5 oz kidney beans

- 2 oz sweet corn

- 3 tablespoons tomato paste

- ½ chili pepper

- 1 ½ tablespoons ground paprika

- ½ teaspoon basil (dried or fresh)

- 7 oz tofu

For the marinade:

- 3 tablespoons soy sauce

- 2 ½ tablespoons olive oil

- ½ teaspoon mustard

- Salt and pepper

- Some water

The Instructions

1. Start with the tofu marinade. Mix the soy sauce with the olive oil and mustard in a

bowl and season with salt and pepper. Crumble the tofu with a fork and mix it with

the marinade. Leave it to soak for at least one hour. You could also marinade the tofu

the night before.

2. Peel and dice the onion and garlic. Rinse the kidney beans. Wash and dice the bel

pepper, tomatoes and the chili pepper.

3. Sauté the onions and garlic in olive oil in a large and deep pan. Add the marinated

tofu and fry it until it's nice and crispy.

4. Add the diced bel pepper, the crushed tomatoes, the fresh tomato pieces, the tomato

paste, the chili pepper and the sweet corn. Add a little water and let simmer over

medium heat for 20 minutes.

5. Season well with the spices and keep on simmering until the chili reaches a nice,

creamy consistency.

6. Serve with some sourdough bread and enjoy!

Recipe 16 - Pesto Presto

Ever wanted to make your own pesto? Now's the time!

The Ingredients (2 servings)

- 1 ¾ oz pine nuts

- 1 ¾ oz walnuts

- ⅓ cup olive oil

- 1 ½ oz basil

- ½ teaspoon salt

- 1 tablespoon nutritional yeast

The Instructions

1. Warm up a frying pan on medium heat. Don't add any oil or fat. Gently roast the

walnuts and pine nuts. Watch out so you don't burn them.

2. Fil the roasted nuts into a high jar and add the basil, salt and olive oil before blending everything with a handheld mixer

(or similar gear). Blend until you have a smooth

paste.

3. Stir in the nutritional yeast to give the pesto some extra creaminess and flavour.

4. Serve with some spaghetti or whatever pasta you like the most (just make sure it

doesn't have eggs in it).

Recipe 17 - Kill it with Millet

Mil et is a real superfood! It contains a lot of good micronutrients and goes wel with a lot of veggies. Just like this:

The Ingredients (2 servings)

- 9 oz mil et

- 3 ½ cups water

- 1 onion

- 1 zucchini

- ½ eggplant

- 1 red bel pepper

- 4 tablespoons olive oil

- 2.8 oz tomato paste

- 2 tablespoons oregano, dried

- 1 oz alfalfa sprouts

- 1 ½ oz roasted hazelnuts

- Salt and pepper

The Instructions

1. Fil a pot with the water and add ½ teaspoon of salt and the mil et. Bring to a boil then reduce to medium heat and let simmer for about 22 minutes. Stir occasionally.

2. Peel and dice the onion. Wash the zucchini and eggplant and cut into smaller bits.

Wash and dice the bel pepper.

3. Heat up about 3 tablespoons of olive oil in a frying pan and gently sweat the

vegetables for about 5 minutes. Add the oregano and tomato paste, then fry for an

additional minute and keep stirring. Season with salt and pepper.

4. Stir in the mil et and season some more.

5. Serve with alfalfa sprouts and hacked hazelnuts sprinkled on top.

6. Enjoy!

Recipe 18 - Ermahgerd Burger

Final y, something familiar! Black beans are great for making patties. Here's how:

The Ingredients (2 servings)

- 1 cup black beans

- ¼ large red onion

- 1 small garlic clove

- ⅓ cup chopped parsley

- ¼ teaspoon salt

- ¼ red chili

- ⅓ cup crushed pumpkin seeds

- 0.5 oz potato flour

- Some vegetable oil for frying

- 2 burger buns of your preference (just make sure they're vegan)

- Some lettuce, tomato, onion and sauces of your preference for the burger

The Instructions

1. Rinse the black beans before mashing them with a fork in a bowl.

2. Combine the mashed beans with the other ingredients. Add the potato flour at the

end.

3. Form two patties and fry them in oil for about 3-4 minutes on each side.

4. Serve with the bread buns and add all the good stuff you'd like on your burger.

5. Enjoy!

Recipe 19 - Oumph my Gawd

What the heck is Oumph? This delicious new soy based product was invented in the North

of Europe and has now made its way from Sweden into US stores. Try it instead of tofu or

other fake meats. My suggestion is to have it in a exotic glass noodle salad.

The Ingredients (2 servings)

For the salad:

- 3.5 oz glass noodles

- 4.5 oz spring onion

- 7 oz kale

- 9 oz carrots

- 5.5 oz sugar snap peas

- 1 small bunch of fresh coriander

- 1 tablespoon rapeseed oil

- 10 oz Oumph

- 8 oz mango, diced

For the dressing:

- ½ red chili pepper

- 1 tablespoon ginger

- 1 garlic clove

- 2 tablespoons rapeseed oil

- ½ teaspoon agave syrup

- 1 lime

The Instructions

1. Prepare and boil the glass noodle according to the instructions on the package.

Afterwards, hold them under cold water to cool them down and place them in a large

bowl

2. Wash the spring onion and cut it in smaller stripes. Wash the kale and take away the

stems before chopping up the leaves. Peel the carrots and grate them. Wash the

sugar snap peas and cut them in half. Wash and chop the coriander. Mix everything

with the drained glass noodles.

3. Chop the red chili pepper into small pieces. Peel and grate the ginger, pressed the

garlic. Mix with oil, agave syrup and lime juice. Add to the noodles and mix everything thoroughly.

4. Heat up some more oil in a frying pan and fry the Oumph pieces for about 4 minutes.

Stir continuously.

5. Serve the glass noodle salad in a bowl and top it off with the magno pieces and the

fried Oumph.

6. Enjoy!

Recipe 20 - Sweet & Chunky

This is a quick and easy one, but it's so yummy!

The Ingredients (2 servings)

- 1 lbs sweet potato

- 10 oz smoked tofu

- vegetable oil

- 4 tablespoons vegan BBQ sauce

- Salt and pepper

The Instructions

1. Preheat the oven to 400°F (200°C).

2. Wash the sweet potato before cutting it into small wedges. Oil and season the

wedges with 2 tablespoons of vegetable oil, salt and pepper. Distribute them evenly

on a baking tray and put it in the oven for about 20 minutes. When the wedges are

soft on the inside and roasted golden on the outside, they are done.

3. Cut the tofu into small stripes. Heat up the remaining oil in a pan and fry the tofu

slices crispy on each side.

4. Serve the tofu and sweet potatoes with your favorite vegan BBQ sauce.

5. Enjoy!

Recipe 21 - Oven-veg-tastic

Simple, simple, simple. Veggies in the oven!

The Ingredients (2 servings)

For the veggies:

- 7 oz sweet potato

- 7 oz zucchini

- 4 carrots

- 2 red onions

- 2 garlic cloves

- 2 tablespoons olive oil

- Salt and pepper

For the dressing:

- 2 tablespoons tahini (sesame paste)

- 4 tablespoons lemon juice

- 2 garlic cloves, pressed

- 4 tablespoons olive oil

- Salt and pepper

The Instructions

1. Preheat the oven to 425°F (220°C).

2. Wash the veggies and peel the ones you'd like without skin (I like my sweet potatoes

with their peel on, others don't. Matter of taste, really). Cut the sweet potatoes,

carrots and zucchini in pinky-thin slices. Quarter the onions. Dice the garlic.

3. Mix all the veggies with oil (except the tomatoes), season them and place them

evenly on an oven tray.

4. Gril the veggies in the oven on a middle level for about 40 minutes until the insides

are soft and the outsides started to get crispy golden. Cut the tomatoes in halves and

add them to the veggies. Gril for another 15 minutes.

5. Mix the tahini, lemon juice, pressed garlic, and 4 tablespoons olive oil to make the

dressing. Season with salt and pepper.

6. Let the veggies cool down a bit before mixing in the dressing. Serve and top off with some roasted sunflower seeds if you like.

7. Enjoy!

Recipe 22 - Keep Calm and Hail Seitan

Don't worry, we won't summon any demons here. Saitan is a protein rich, wheat-based meat replacement. The largest part of Seitan is actual y Gluten, so if you're intolerant, better stay away from this recipe. While you can buy Seitan ready-made, I'm going to show you how to

make it yourself. In this specific recipe I'l show you how to make seitan sausages.

The Ingredients (2 servings)

For the sausages:

- 5 oz gluten

- 2 tablespoons chickpea flour

- 4 tablespoons nutritional yeast

- 2 tablespoons dried marjoram

- 1 teaspoon onion powder

- ½ teaspoon ground black pepper

- 1 teaspoon salt

- 2.3 oz smoked tofu

- 2 garlic cloves, pressed

- 1 cup water

For the sauce:

- ½ lbs ketchup

- ¼ cups water

- 1 tablespoon soy sauce

- 2 tablespoons curry powder

- ½ teaspoon cayenne pepper, ground

The Instructions

1. Preheat the oven to 400°F (200°C)

2. Mix the gluten, chickpea flour, nutritional yeast, marjoram, onion powder, salt and

pepper. Mash the smoked tofu into a paste and add it to the gluten mix with the pressed garlic and water. Knead everything to a dough. Let it rest for a couple of

minutes, the knead some more.

3. Form the dough into 4 sausages. Roll every sausage tightly in some aluminium foil

and bake for about 25 minutes in the oven.

4. For the sauce add all ingredients in a pot. Heat up and let simmer for about 1 minute.

5. Cut the sausages into pieces and serve with the sauce.

6. Enjoy your German style "curry sausage" (Surprise!)

The Recipes

Part III: Dinner

Recipe 23 - Hummus

It's getting late. Dinner time! Let's stay the evening with a true classic and my favorite food of all time. Goes perfect with anything. Especially as a dip.

The Ingredients (1 bowl)

- 8 oz of pre-boiled chickpeas (usually come canned)

- Some water

- 2 tablespoons macadamia oil (olive oil is fine too)

- 1 garlic clove

- 1 teaspoon lemon juice

- 1 teaspoon tahini (sesame paste)

- 1 teaspoon chili powder

- 1 teaspoon ground paprika powder (mild)

- Some salt and pepper

- Optional: fresh coriander

The Instructions

1. Drain the chickpeas but keep some of the water from the can or pack in a separate

glass. Fil the chickpeas in a jar or high bowl you're gonna mix the hummus in.

2. Hack the garlic and add it to the chickpeas with the oil, the lemon juice, the tahini, and the spices.

3. Blend everything with a handheld mixer (or similar devices) and slowly add some

water until the hummus is nice and creamy. You can decide how creamy or thick the

hummus should turn out, but don't make it too runny. Fresh coriander is optional, but

I recommend it.

4. Tip: If you let the hummus stand in the fridge overnight, the taste wil be even

better and more intense the next day. Nom!

5. Serve with oven veggies or fresh bread. I have hummus with everything.

6. Enjoy your creamy goodness!

Recipe 24 - SOUPer Green

What's hot and green and fits into a bowl?

The Ingredients (2 bowls)

- 1 smaller onion

- 1 garlic clove

- 1 tablespoon rapeseed oil

- 1 ⅓ cups vegetable broth

- ½ cup coconut cream

- 7 oz spinach, chopped

- 3 oz green peas

- Salt and pepper

The Instructions

1. Peel and dice the onion and garlic. Sauté in a large pot with some oil. Fil in the broth and coconut cream. Bring to a boil.

2. Add the spinach, peas and season with a little salt and pepper. Let it simmer a while before blending everything with a handheld mixer.

3. Serve with some fresh parsley and nice bread.

4. Enjoy!

Recipe 25 - Quinoa Patties

Quinoa is another superfood and already the Incas knew of its benefits. Here's how you

make some yummy patties with it.

The Ingredients (2 servings)

• 7 oz quinoa

- 2 red onions

- 1 bunch of parsley

- 2 teaspoons mustard

- 2 teaspoons locust bean gum (thickening agent)

- 1 teaspoon sweet paprika powder

- 3-4 tablespoons olive oil

- Salt and pepper

The Instructions

1. Start cooking the quinoa in a large pot. Boil until the shel s break open and the

quinoa is nice and soft. Drain afterwards so that only the cooked quinoa is left.

2. Peel and cut the onions into fine cubes. Wash the parsley and chop the leaves.

3. Combine the quinoa with the locust bean gum, mustard, parsley, onions and sweet

paprika powder. Knead everything into a thick mass (just like you would with real

meat patties). Season with salt and pepper.

4. Form about 10 smaller patties and fry them in a pan with the olive oil over medium

heat. Fry each side for about 4 minutes until roasted golden.

5. Serve with dip and sides of your choosing (Did I hear Hummus?)

6. Enjoy!

Recipe 26 - Spaghetti Volognese

Another simple classic and kids favorite made vegan.

The Ingredients (2 servings)

• 5 ½ oz of spaghetti

• ½ large onion

- 1 garlic clove

- ¼ carrot

- ⅛ cup olive oil

- 1 teaspoon dried oregano

- 1 teaspoon dried basil

- 4 oz hard tofu

- 2 tablespoons tomato paste

- 1 tablespoon sugar

- 1 tärningar grönsaksbuljong

- 7 oz crushed tomatoes

The Instructions

1. Cook the spaghetti according to the instructions on the package (some pasta takes a

few minutes longer than others).

2. Dice the garlic and onion, and grate the carrot.

3. Crush the tofu into small crumbs with a fork.

4. Heat up a frying pan and gently roast the garlic, onion and carrot. Add the dried basil and oregano.

5. Add the crumbled tofu, the tomato paste and sugar. Fry for about 3 minutes and stir

constantly.

6. Add the crushed tomatoes and stir the sauce before letting it cook on low heat for

another 3 minutes.

7. Serve the spaghetti with the sauce and add some fresh basil for decoration and extra

taste.

8. Enjoy!

Recipe 27 - SOUPer Red

More soups for everyone!

The Ingredients (2 bowls)

- ½ onion

- 2 teaspoons vegetable oil

- 2 cups vegetable broth

- a little less than ½ cup red lentils

- 2 teaspoons ground paprika (mild)

- 14 oz crushed tomatoes (canned)

- 2 garlic cloves

- 2 teaspoons red wine vinegar

- ½ teaspoon ground thyme

- ½ teaspoon ground basil

- 1 teaspoon salt

The Instructions

1. Peel and dice the onion. Sauté in a pot with the oil.

2. Add the broth, lentils, crushed tomatoes and the ground paprika.

3. Place a lid on the pot and let everything cook for about 15 minutes. Add the pressed

garlic and season soup with the additional spices and salt.

4. Enjoy with some nice bread!

Recipe 28 - Garlic Schmarlic

This one's for the lazy folks. It's so ridiculously easy, it hurts a bit. I love to indulge in garlic butter, though, so I need to share this with you!

The Ingredients

● ½ cup vegan margarine or vegan spread

● 2 garlic cloves

● 2 tablespoons of freshly chopped chives or parsley

• Salt and pepper

The Instructions

1. Leave the margarine out for a while so it softens in room temperature.

2. Peel and chop the garlic into tiny bits.

3. Mix the garlic and chives/parsley with the margarine/spread, then season with salt

and pepper.

4. That's basically it. Easy, right?

5. Enjoy with bread or gril ed corn or whatever floats your boat. Nom!

Recipe 29 - Vegan BBQ? Vegan BBQ!

The biggest temptation to eat meat again always comes in three letters: BBQ. When your

friends a firing up the barbie and the smell of meat and fat and spices fil s the air, all you can think of is that juicy burger. But don't panic! There are alternatives for you, if you want to stay the course.

The Ingredients (1 serving)

- 2 cobs of corn

- 2 onions

- 1 pack of smoked tofu

- 1 red bel pepper

- 1 zucchini

- 2 tablespoons olive oil

- Vegan garlic butter (see above)

- Salt and pepper

The Instructions

1. The corn: slap some vegan garlic butter on the cobs and put them on the BBQ. Turn

regularly.

2. The veggie skewers: Cut the onions in quarters. Dice the tofu. Cut smaller wedges

out of the bel pepper. Slice the zucchini (about a finger wide). Put the veggies on two

metal BBQ skewers. Marinade the veggies with the oil and season with salt and

pepper. Gril them until roasted golden. Serve with some vegan BBQ sauce or

whatever floats your boat.

3. Enjoy!

Recipe 30 - Quinoa Salad

Quinoa is not only good as patties, but also in salads!

The Ingredients (2 servings)

- 7 oz of quinoa

- 1 red bel pepper

- 1 avocado

- 3 oz cherry tomatoes

- 1 salad onion

- 1 tablespoon olive oil

- 1 tablespoon lime juice

- 1 teaspoon sambal oelek

- Salt and pepper

- 1 bunch of fresh parsley

The Instructions

1. Fil a pot with about 5 cups of water. Add a pinch of salt. Boil the quinoa until the shel s broke open and the seeds have softened. Pour out the water that's left in the

pot and let the quinoa drip in a strainer.

2. Chop the salad onion is small slices. Cut the tomatoes and the avocado in half. Whas

and dice the bel pepper. Cut the "meat" of the avocado in cubes.

3. Chop some of the parsley and mix it with the olive oil, lime juice, sambal oelek, salt and pepper. Mix this dressing with the quinoa and add the veggies.

4. Serve with fresh parsley leaves on top.

5. Enjoy!

Recipe 31 - Rock & Summer Roll

Summer rolls, also known as vietnamese spring rolls, are a hit at every dinner party and can be made vegan easily!

The Ingredients (All You Can Eat)

For the rolls:

• Rice paper wrappers (round and dry)

• Glass noodles

• Red bel peppers

- Salad onions

- Carrots

- Cucumbers

- Tofu

- Fresh parsley, coriander

For the peanut sauce:

- ¼ cup creamy peanut butter

- 13.5 oz of coconut milk (canned)

- 1 tablespoon soy sauce

- 1 teaspoon red curry paste

- Optional: chili flakes

The Instructions

1. Preheat the oven to 400°F (200°C). Bake the tofu in finger-wide strips until golden.

2. While the tofu is in the oven, cut all vegetables into very thin strips. Also cook

the glass noodles according to the instructions on the packaging.

3. For the sauce: combine all ingredients in a saucepan over medium heat. Stir

occasionally while cooking for a few minutes.

4. Serving the rice paper rol s: have a deep and wide plate on the table and fil it with hot water (not so hot that you burn your fingers). For every roll, put a rice paper

wrapper into the water and let it soak until it's soft and flexible. This shouldn't take

more than a minute. Put the rice paper roll on a plate and add all the good stuff you

want in your spring roll. Wrap it into a nice little package of yummy goodness. Have

the peanut sauce either as a dip or inside the roll.

5. Enjoy and share with friends!

Recipe 32 - Souper Creamy

Enough of red and green. Have some cream!

The Ingredients (2 bowls)

- 4.5 oz mushrooms

- ¼ onion

- ½ garlic cloves

- 2 cups of vegetable broth

- 2 tablespoons olive oil

- 1 tablespoon wheat flour

- 1 pinch of chili flakes

- 1 teaspoon lemon juice

- 1 teaspoon mixed herbs, chopped (parsley, basil etc.)

- Salt and pepper

- 1 salad onion

- ½ cup coconut cream

The Instructions

1. Peel and dice onion, and press the garlic. Wash and cut the mushrooms into smaller

pieces.

2. Fry the onion, garlic and mushrooms in a large pot with the olive oil for about 5

minutes.

3. Add the flour and stir well. Add the vegetable broth, salt, pepper and chiliflakes, the lemon juice and the rest of the chosen spices. Stir well.

4. Let it boil for about 10 minutes. Stir occasionally.

5. Blend the soup with a handheld electric mixer.

6. Wash and cut the salad onion into slices. Add them and the coconut cream to the

soup and bring to a final boil.

7. Serve and enjoy with some nice bread!

Recipe 33 - It's a wrap!

Wow, you made it to the last recipe. Great success. Let's close with an easy one. Yummy

supper wraps for the win!

The Ingredients (2 wraps)

- 2 tortil a wraps

- 4 tablespoons vegan spread or margarine

- 1 handful of lettuce or other salad

- 2 avocados

- 2 red-skinned radishes

- A few pickled red onion

- Salt and pepper

- Fresh parsley

The Instructions

1. Cut the avocado meat in thinner slices. Also slice the radishes.

2. Spread some margarine on the wrap. Add the salad, avocado slices, radish slices

and pickled onion. Season with a little salt and pepper and top off with some fresh

parsley.

3. Roll up and enjoy!

Part 2

Introduction

Vegan Mastery Cookbook: Simple Chinese Vegan Recipes to Cook at Home is your one-stop source for creating the perfect Chinese appetizers, entrees and desserts for your friends and family.

Inside you will be treated to a wide selection of vegan Chinese recipes, making it easy to satisfy all preferences. There are recipes that will suit every palate on any occasion whether it is fall, spring, summer, or winter.

Recipes include:

Vegan Hot and Sour Soup

"Egg" Drop Soup

Steamed Dumplings

Spicy Sesame Peanut Noodles

"Beef" and Broccoli Stir Fry

Vegan Orange Chicken

8 Treasure Rice Pudding

Vegan Almond Cookies

Vegan Sweet and Sour "Chicken"

And more...

Celebrate the joy of plant-based cuisine with Vegan Mastery Cookbook: Simple Chinese Vegan Recipes to Cook at Home.

Thanks again for downloading this book. I hope you enjoy it!

Vegan "Egg" Drop Soup

Ingredients

2 Cups Vegetable Broth

5 Oz Finely Sliced Packet of Silken Tofu

4 Shitake Mushrooms-sliced thin

1/2Inch Piece of Ginger Finely Grated

1 Garlic Clove-finely grated

1 Tablespoon Rice Wine Vinegar

1 Teaspoon Sesame Oil

1 Stalk of Finely Diced Scallion

½ Tablespoon Soy Sauce (or Tamari Sauce)

Sriracha to Taste

Preparation

In a sauce pan, add all ingredients except tofu and scallions. Bring to a boil.

Next, add tofu slowly and stir. Reduce to a simmer.

Check for seasoning. If soup needs flavor add more Soy Sauce or Tamari Sauce.

Add scallions and serve!

Vegan Hot and Sour Soup

Ingredients

8-ounce Chinese Noodles (follow instructions on package)

2 Tablespoons Sunflower Oil or Canola Oil

2 Garlic Cloves-minced

½ Teaspoon Fresh Ginger-minced

½ Teaspoon Dried Chili Flakes

4 Cups Vegetable Broth

1 Tablespoon Tamari Sauce or Soy Sauce

¼ Teaspoon Ground White Pepper

3 Tablespoons Chinese Black Vinegar (find at local Asian markets)

½ Teaspoon Toasted Sesame Oil

3 Tablespoons Potato Starch

¼ Cup Bok Choy-chopped

¼ Cup Fresh Shiitake Mushrooms-hard stems removed

1 Small Carrot-julienned

3-ounce Firm Tofu-diced into 1/2-inch cubes

2 Medium Scallions-finely chopped

1 Tablespoon Cilantro-chopped

Preparation

Boil Chinese noodles according to package instructions. After noodles are cooked, remove nooldes from the pot and place them in a tray full of cold water. Set aside.

In a large pot, heat oil, and sauté garlic and ginger on medium heat until fragrant. Add dried chili flakes. Then, pour in broth.

Next, add white pepper, sesame oil, Chinese black vinegar, and soy sauce into the pot and stir for 3 minutes.

Next, add all vegetables & tofu and allow to cook for 8-10 minutes.

Meanwhile, in a separate bowl, dissolve starch in ½ cup cold water until smooth and then add to soup while it is boiling. Stir continually.

Prepare your cooked noodles in serving bowls. Add the soup to the serving bowls.

Garnish with cilantro and green onions and serve!

Chinese "Chicken" Salad

Ingredients

2 packages vegan "chicken" strips-diced

1 Head of Lettuce-cut into small piece

4 Green Onions-diced thin

4 Celery Stalks-sliced thin

1/2 Cup Walnuts-chopped

2 Tablespoons Toasted Sesame Seeds

6 Ounces Chinese Noodles-heated briefly to crisp

6 Tablespoons Seasoned Rice Vinegar

4 Tablespoons White Sugar or Stevia

1 Teaspoon Salt

1/2 Cup Peanut Oil

Preparation

In a large salad bowl, combine "chicken" strips, lettuce, green onion, nuts, celery, seeds and noodles. Mix together. and set aside.

Dressing Preparation: Add vinegar into a small bowl. Dissolve sugar and salt in vinegar then add oil. Beat well.

Add dressing to salad and toss.

Serve and enjoy!

Steamed Dumplings

Ingredients

1/2 Cup Mushrooms-finely chopped

1/2 cup Grated Carrots

1/2 Cup Cabbage-shredded

2 Tablespoon Red Pepper-finely chopped

2 Tablespoon Onion-finely chopped

2 Teaspoons Fresh Ginger-minced

1 Tablespoon Soy Sauce or Tamari Sauce

1 Tablespoon Sesame Oil

Salt and pepper-to taste

Approximately 40 small dumpling wrapper

Preparation

In a large bowl, combine carrots, mushrooms, cabbage, red pepper, onion, ginger, soy sauce (or tamari sauce), and sesame oil. Stir and season with salt and pepper.

Form the dumplings by individually placing the wrappers on a dry working surface. Place 1 teaspoon of vegetable mixture in the center of the wrapper. Next, wet the edges of the wrapper with water and proceed to fold one side over and pinch edges until sealed. Repeat until all of the filling is gone.

Next, bring approximately half inch of water to a simmer over medium heat. In a steamer, place as many dumplings as possible without them touching each other. Cover and steam for 10 to 12 minutes. Repeat until all dumplings are cooked.

Serve dumplings hot with a side of hoisin sauce or sauce of your choice.

Vegan Fried Rice

Ingredients

2 cups rice

3 Tablespoons Vegetable Oil

¾ Cup Green Beans-finely chopped

2 Carrots-finely chopped

1 Onion-sliced

¾ Cups Finely Chopped Cabbage

1 Teaspoon Garlic-finely chopped

2 Tablespoons Tamari Sauce or Soy Sauce

1 Tablespoon Vinegar

Salt and Pepper-to taste

Preparation

Cook rice according to directions on package. Next, heat oil in large pan and stir fry all of the chopped vegetables. Cook for 3 – 5 minutes. Add salt and pepper to taste.

Add cooked rice to vegetables and mix. Next, add soy sauce and vinegar. Cook the fried rice for approximately 3 minutes.

Serve fried rice and enjoy!

Ginger Teriyaki Noodles

Ingredients

2 Tablespoons Teriyaki Sauce

2 Tablespoons Soy Sauce

2 Tablespoons Wine Vinegar

2 Tablespoons Ground Ginger

2 Celery Stalks-diced

1 Carrot-diced

½ Onion-diced

2/3 Cup Snow Peas

4 Scallions-sliced

3 Tablespoons Olive Oil

1 Tablespoon Sesame Oil

1 Pound Chinese-Style Noodles or Lo Mein Noodles

Preparation

Mix the soy sauce, teriyaki sauce, vinegar and ginger together and set aside.

Then, cook the Chinese noodles until soft, about 6 to 8 minutes. Drain well.

In a large wok, sautee the vegetables in 2 tablespoons of the olive oil for 4 to 5 minutes until tender.

Add remaining oil and the teriyaki and soy sauce mixture to the skillet. Next, add the Chinese noodles. Allow to cook for another 6 minutes, stirring continuously.

Serve and enjoy!

Vegan Chinese Noodles

Ingredients

1 Pound Asian Noodles or Spaghetti

5 Green Onions-sliced

4 Garlic Cloves-minced

½ Teaspoon Olive Oil

½ Cup Vegetable Broth

1/ Teaspoon Cornstarch

1/3 Cup Soy Sauce or Tamari Sauce

2 Tablespoons Ketchup

1 Tablespoon Vinegar

1 Tablespoon Chili Sauce (Sriracha or Hot Sauce)

1 Teaspoon Sugar or Stevia

1/3 Cup Peanuts

1 Cucumber-sliced thin

Preparation

First, cook the spaghetti or Asian noodles according to the instructions on the package.

Next, in a large wok, sautee the garlic and green onions for two minutes. Next, add the remaining ingredients (except the peanuts and cucumber) and whisk together.

Then, add the cucumber, peanuts, and noodles, stirring well. Cook until heated all the way through.

Plate and serve!

Chinese Pear and Avocado Bowl

Ingredients

½ Avocado-pitted, peeled, and diced

1 15-oz. Can of Chickpeas-drained

1 Asian pear (med-sized)-cored and sliced thin

2 celery Stalks-chopped

1 Cup Cucumber-diced

1 Jalapeño Chili (small)-stemmed, seeded, and minced

¼ Cup Cilantro-chopped

1 Tablespoon Canola Oil

2 Tablespoons Fresh Lime Juice

Preparation

Combine all ingredients into a bowl. Season with salt and pepper.

Serve and enjoy!

Spicy Sesame Peanut Noodles

Ingredients

¼ Cup Soy Sauce or Tamari Sauce

2/3 Cup Peanut Butter

3 Garlic Cloves-minced

2 Green Onions-diced

2 Tablespoons Sesame Oil

½ Teaspoon Ginger Powder

½ Teaspoon Cayenne Pepper Powder

1 Lime-juiced

½ Pound Asian Noodles or Spaghetti

2 Tablespoons Sesame Seeds

Preparation

First, cook noodles according to the package directions. Heat pan to low heat and add all ingredients (except noodles and sesame seeds). Stir together carefully.

Next, pour the sauce that is in the pan over the noodles gently tossing to combine. Add the sesame seeds on top.

Serve hot or cold and enjoy!

Vegetable Lo Mein

Ingredients

8 Ounces of Udon or Soba Noodles

5 Green Onions

3 Garlic Cloves-minced

1 ½ Tablespoons Fresh Ginger-grated

½ Teaspoon Red Pepper Flakes

1 Cup Mushrooms-sliced

1 Handful Snow Peas

1 Can Bamboo Shoots-drained

2 Yellow Squash-thinly sliced

3 Carrots-thinly sliced

½ Cup Vegetable Broth

1 ½ Teaspoon Salt

Lo Mein Sauce **Ingredients**

2 Teaspoons Rice Vinegar

4 Tablespoons Soy Sauce or Tamari Sauce

¼ Teaspoon Ground Ginger

¼ Teaspoon Garlic Powder

½ Teaspoon Agave Nectar

½ Teaspoon Hot Sauce (i.e. Sriracha)

½ Teaspoon Vegetable Oil

Preparation

First, prepare the noodles according to the package instructions.

Next, prepare the sauce by cooking sauce ingredients over low heat for a few minutes until all ingredients are blended well. In a hot pan/wok, add the broth and stir fry the veggies until tender. Next, add the cooked noodles to the wok/pan. Stir all ingredients together. Then, pour the Lo Mein sauce over the top and fry a few minutes longer stirring continuously.

Plate the dish, sprinkle with minced dark green section of onions, and serve!

Eggplant and Potato Chinese Dish

Ingredients

1 Eggplant-sliced into cubes
1 Green Pepper-diced
1 Potato-peeled and cut into squares
2 Garlic Cloves-chopped
1 Tablespoon of Soy Sauce or Tamari Sauce
Salt, sugar/Stevia, Oil

Preparation

First choose an eggplant that is heavy and firm with an even dark color.

Pat the eggplant dry with a paper towel before cooking it. Slice and salt the eggplant.

There are dozens of ways to cook the eggplant. Options include deep-frying, grilling, baking, steaming, sauté, pickling, etc. Keep in mind that the eggplant soaks up oil like a sponge, especially good olive oil.

Saute the potatoes and eggplant separately in a pan with oil until each golden brown. Remove each and drain.

Next, stir-fry the green peppers with a tablespoon of oil in a separate pan for a few minutes.

Add the cooked eggplant and potatoes to the green peppers, along with the soy sauce or tamari sauce, chopped garlic, salt and a pinch of sugar/stevia.

Continue to stir fry for a few minutes then remove from heat.

Serve hot and enjoy!

Vegan Orange Chicken

Ingredients

1 package of Gardein Mandarin Orange Chick'n

1 "boil in a bag" rice (brown or wild)

2 Tablespoons Hoisin Sauce

Assorted Vegetables-fresh or frozen stir-fry style

¼ Cup Sweet Chili Sauce

2 Tablespoons Olive Oil

Preparation

First, boil rice then set aside. Then, place Gardein sauce packet in warm water to thaw and set aside.

Next, heat olive oil in a pan on medium high and add "chick'n" to pan and cook until slightly crisp.

Add assorted vegetables to the same pan-cook until slightly crisp and tender.

Next, add Gardein sauce to the chicken & vegetables and mix well. Then, add the hoisin sauce & sweet chili sauce to the mixture.

Place mixture over rice and serve!

Kung Pao "Chicken" & Vegetables

Ingredients

¾ Cup Diced Carrots

8 Ounces Mushrooms-sliced

¾ Cup Celery-sliced

¾ Cup Onion-diced

1 package of vegan "chicken"

8 Ounces Water Chestnuts-diced

½ Cup Dry Roasted Peanuts (optional)

3 Garlic Cloves-minced

3 Stalks Bok Choy-diced

3 Teaspoons Rice Wine/Sake

3 Teaspoons Soy Sauce or Tamari

2 Teaspoons Rice Vinegar

2 Teaspoons Cornstarch in ¼ Cup Water

Sriracha (hot sauce) to taste

Preparation

Place the sliced mushrooms in a pan and stir until mushrooms are released of their liquid. Add celery, carrots, and onions and cook until colors of vegetables brighten. Next, add peanuts (optional), water chestnuts, Bok Choy, and garlic and cook until heated all the way through.

In a separate bowl, mix together the soy sauce (or tamari sauce), rice vinegar, and rice wine. Then, pour over the vegetables, mix together, and cook until mix bubbles slightly. Then, add the cornstarch that has been dissolved in water to thicken the sauce.

Add the Sriracha to taste and serve over rice!

"Chicken" and Broccoli

Ingredients

2 Tablespoons Sesame Oil

6 Garlic Cloves-minced

¼ Cup Soy Sauce or Tamari Sauce

1-1/2 Cups Vegetable Broth

¼ Cup Mirin (sweet rice wine)

1 Tablespoon Agave

½ Teaspoon Hoisin Sauce

2 Teaspoons Cornstarch

2 Packages Vegan Chicken-diced

Brown or White Rice "Boil in a Bag"

Preparation

Prepare the rice according to package instructions and set aside.

Then, blanch the broccoli (cook in boiling water for a few minutes). Drain broccoli and run under cold water so it stays bright green.

Heat sesame oil in a large pan. Next, add the garlic and cook until lightly browned.

Add soy sauce (or tamari sauce), vegetable broth, mirin, hoisin sauce, and agave, then stir to combine. Cook for approximately seven minutes.

Then, mix a small amount of the sauce with the corn starch to make a slurry. Then add it to the sauce. Next, add the vegan chicken and cook, stirring continuously, until cooked all the way through.

Next, add in the broccoli and stir to combine.

Serve with rice and enjoy!

"Beef" and Broccoli Stir Fry

Ingredients

4 Ounces Tempeh-cut into 1/2-inch pieces

1/4 Cup Soy Sauce or Tamari Sauce

1 Tablespoon Rice Vinegar

3 Garlic Cloves-minced

2 Teaspoons Fresh Ginger-peeled and minced

1 Pinch Dried Crushed Red Pepper

12 Ounces Broccoli-stems peeled and cut into 1/2-inch pieces & florets cut into 1-inch pieces

2 Tablespoons Water

1 Teaspoon Agave

1 Teaspoon Cornstarch

1 Tablespoon Vegetable Oil

1/2 Cup Red Bell Pepper-chopped

2 Tablespoons Green Onion-thinly sliced

Preparation

Stir ginger, tempeh, soy sauce, vinegar, garlic, and crushed red pepper and chopped red bell pepper in a bowl and mix ingredients. Allow to marinate for one hour at room temperature.

Next, steam the broccoli for approximately 3 minutes and set aside. Then, strain the marinade from tempeh into small bowl and set the tempeh aside.

Whisk the 2 tablespoons water, agave and cornstarch into marinade.

Next, heat oil in large pan over high heat. Add the marinated bell pepper and tempeh and cook for 4 minutes. Add broccoli and marinade mixture and sauté until broccoli is heated through for approximately 3 minutes. Transfer to bowl.

Plate, top with green onion, and serve!

Chicken and Mushroom Stir Fry

Ingredients

2 Packages of Vegan "Chicken"

½ Pound Mushrooms (med-sized)

2 Garlic Cloves

1 ½ Tablespoons Vegetable Oil for cooking

1 Teaspoon Sesame Oil

Salt and Pepper-to taste

3 Tablespoons Soy Sauce or Tamari Sauce

1 Tablespoon Cornstarch

1 Teaspoon Sugar

Preparation

First, if vegan chicken is not already sliced, slice into thin pieces. Next, in a bowl, combine "chicken" pieces with the marinade ingredients. Mix together and set aside.

Wash the mushrooms and slice into ¼ inch thin pieces. Then, crush, peel, and finely chop the garlic. Heat 1 tablespoon oil in a pan over medium-high heat. When oil is hot, add the marinated vegan chicken into pan. Cook and stir for approximately 3 minutes until the "chicken" is just about cooked through. Transfer "chicken" onto a plate or bowl and set aside. Add ½ tablespoon oil into the pan. Brown the garlic for a few seconds then add the sliced mushrooms, salt and pepper to pan. Cook and stir the mushrooms for about 1 to 2 minutes until the mushrooms are soft. Add the cooked chicken back into the pan and mix. Add sesame oil and cook for a few seconds longer.

Serve dish hot and enjoy!

Vegan Sweet and Sour "Chicken"

2 Packages Vegan "Chicken" Strips-cut into bite-sized pieces

1 Tablespoon Arrowroot Powder

2 Tablespoons Tamari Sauce or Soy Sauce

2 Tablespoons Oil

2 Garlic Cloves-minced

2 Teaspoons Fresh Ginger-grated

2 Bell Peppers-chopped

8 Ounces Pineapple Chunks

½ Onion (medium-sized)-chopped

2 Garlic Cloves-minced

2 Teaspoons Fresh Ginger-grated

Extra Juice from the Pineapple (can or package)

⅓ Cup Ketchup

¼ Cup Brown Rice Vinegar

¼ Cup Stevia or Sugar

2 Tablespoons Tamari Sauce or Soy Sauce

2 Teaspoon Arrowroot Powder

¼ Cup Water

Preparation

To prepare the marinade: In a bowl, combine the vegan chicken strips, arrowroot powder and tamari or soy sauce and mix. Allow to marinate for at least 30 minutes.

To make the Sweet and Sour Sauce: In a saucepan over medium heat, add the onions and cook 2 minutes until softened. Then, add the garlic and ginger stirring for approximately 30 seconds. Next, add the pineapple juice, ketchup, tamari sauce or soy sauce, brown rice vinegar, and the sugar/Stevia. Bring to a simmer and cook, stirring occasionally, for approximately 3-4 minutes. In a separate bowl, mix the arrowroot and water until smooth. Then, add to the sauce and bring to a boil. Allow to cook for 1 minute then turn off heat and set aside.

To make the Sweet and Sour "Chicken": Heat oil in a pan over med-heat. Add the vegan chicken strips to the pan and cook (turn once) until crisp and slightly browned for approximately 4-5 minutes. Add additional oil to the pan if needed and cook the garlic and ginger for 2 minutes until softened stirring continuously and tossing to coat the vegan chicken strips. Then, add the bell peppers and pineapple chunks. Cook until the pineapple is slightly crisp and pepper are tender for approximately 3-4 minutes.

Next, stir in the sweet and sour sauce mixture into the pan and coat all vegan chicken strips and veggies. Bring to a boil and allow to cook until sauce is thick for approximately 2 minutes.

Serve with rice and enjoy!

8 TREASURE RICE PUDDING

The traditional Chinese New Year rice pudding dish Americanized and Veganized!

Ingredients

2 cups forbidden rice

3/4 cups dried fruit; prunes, apricots, cherries, etc.

1/2 cup adzuki beans (For optimal heath, adzuki beans should be spouted and slow cooked, however, canned beans will work for this recipe.)

1/2 cup water

1/4 vanilla bean

1/4 tsp cinnamon

Topping Ingredient

1 Can Coconut Cream or Coconut Vanilla Ice Cream

Preparation

Rinse forbidden rice for approximately 2 minutes.

Cook forbidden rice according to package instructions.

Next, blend up beans, dried fruit, and water to make a fruit and bean paste.

Then, add the fruit and bean paste to the rice and stir ingredients.

Form rice by packing it down with a spoon in a large bowl. Optional: Create layers with nuts, fresh fruit, caramel, coconut shreds etc.

Top with the coconut cream or coconut vanilla ice cream and serve!

Vegan Almond Cookies

Ingredients

1 Cup Shortening

¼ Teaspoon Salt

3 Cups Flour

1 Teaspoon Baking Soda

¼ Cup Soymilk

1 Cup Sugar or Stevia

2 Teaspoons Almond Extract

Blanched Almonds

Preparation

Cut shortening into the dry ingredients(salt, flour, baking soda, sugar or Stevia). Then, add soy milk and almond extract and mix well. Knead until soft.

Next, form into balls the size of a walnut. Flatten slightly with hand and place on cookie sheet. Press a blanched almond on each cookie.

Bake at 350 for 10 to 15 minutes (watching constantly to not overcook).

Serve to guests and enjoy!

Conclusion

Thank you again for downloading this book!

I hope this book was able to help you to create simple and delicious Chinese vegan recipes to enjoy at home.

About the Author

Rusty Bond is author of several cookbooks on Vegan diet. He has written research papers on the topic and currently lives in California.

www.ingramcontent.com/pod-product-compliance
Lightning Source LLC
Chambersburg PA
CBHW061540050726
47593CB00002B/849